FACE FITNESS

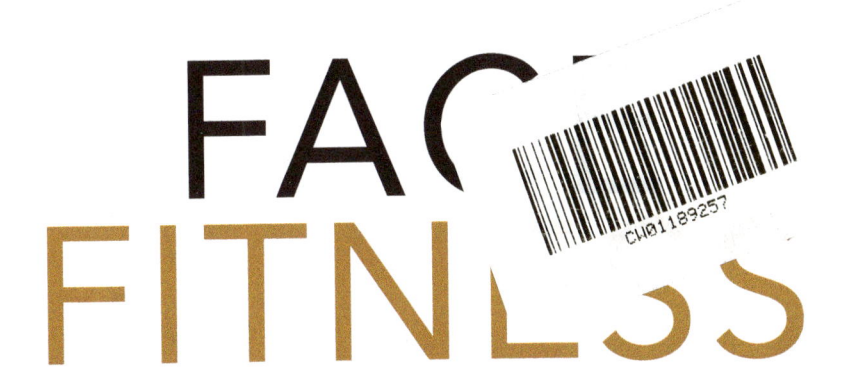

THE 10 MINUTE FACE LIFT

Take *10* Years off Your face

GREGORY LANDSMAN

The Beauty Advisor

This edition published by:

Hill of Content Publishing in Australia
hillofcontentpublishing.com
office@hillofcontentpublishing.com
Correspondence: PO Box 24 East Melbourne 8002 Australia
Distribution: 77 Connaught Road Central Hong Kong

Copyright © 2009 Gregory Landsman
Reprinted 2011, 2018

All rights reserved. No part of this publication may be reproduced, stored in a retrieval system or transmitted in any form by any means without the prior permission of the copyright owner. Enquiries should be made to the publisher.

Every effort has been made to ensure that this book is free from error or omissions. However, the Publisher, the Author, the Editor or their respective employees or agents, shall not accept responsibility for injury, loss or damage occasioned to any person acting or refraining from action as a result of material in this book whether or not such injury, loss or damage is in any way due to any negligent act or omission, breach of duty or default on the part of the Publisher, the Author, the Editor, or their respective employees or agents.

The Author, the Publisher, the Editor and their respective employees or agents do not accept any responsibility for the actions of any person - actions which are related in any way to information contained in this book.

The moral rights of the author have been asserted.

ISBN: 978-0-6482892-5-8

Author: Landsman, Gregory.

Title: Face Fitness : 10 minute face lift / Gregory Landsman.

Design and layout: Jo Hunt

If you want to

TIGHTEN, TONE

and enjoy a

glowing complexion

then

FACE FITNESS

shows you that your

BEAUTY

is in your hands.

TAKE 10 YEARS OFF

Face Fitness is a natural face lift that can take ten years off your face.

All it takes is ten minutes a day to retain or regain a fresh, healthy and younger looking face.

While travelling in India I crossed paths with an amazing seventy-eight-year-old woman who taught me that our genes are not our destiny and that the way our faces age is literally in our hands.

The day she took my hands and clasped them in her own, I knew she would teach me something that would stay with me forever.

What this learned woman shared with me was an ancient Indian treatment that dates back several thousands of years. Having been passed down through her family, it told a story of ancient wisdom steeped in a true understanding of the human form and how to maintain a youthful appearance by keeping the facial muscles fit and skin firm.

This is why I called this program **Face Fitness!**

What I will show you is a powerful and genuine alternative to a surgical face lift that gets results without the $30,000 price tag. It will help you retain and regain a vibrant face without nipping, tucking, sucking and plucking the skin or the facial muscles.

Face Fitness will show you how to:

- Drain toxins that age the skin
- Prevent and reduce wrinkles without anaesthetic
- Sculpt and reshape the face without pain
- Minimise lines around the mouth without collagen
- Lift sagging skin without stitches
- Reduce crow's feet and the folds in the upper and lower eyelids without a surgeon
- Minimise a double chin without cutting
- Tighten jowls and loose skin on the neck without the expense
- Plump up hollow cheeks without face fillers
- Oxygenate the blood to give your skin a lasting healthy glow as well as
- How to eat your way to great skin with the 5 Day Skin Firming Diet

Face Fitness is about conditioning the face in a way that will naturally outlast any surgical face lift or artificial face fillers. This is not only a correction technique for wrinkles and sagging muscles, but a means of prevention as well.

Since learning these techniques I have practised them daily and used them in my career for many years. As I worked with Supermodels, Super mothers and Superstars I shared numerous routines, taking great satisfaction as I watched them impact on each person's face. There is no doubt that if practised consistently this program will not only improve tone, but the overall look of the face.

In a world where so much emphasis is placed on the way we look, where we have all experienced the mental anxiety that sits on our faces, we need a way to keep our faces fresh and healthy, and our minds calm as we journey through the world.

A key part of taking the pressure off comes from understanding that while we all want to look as good as we can for as long as we can, in truth we touch people in a very small way with our looks. Mostly we touch them through acts of kindness and the sharing of our humanity.

My personal philosophy on **B.E.A.U.T.Y.** is…

B alance in our life unfolds from the inside out.

E nthusiasm lies within the way we think and feel about ourselves.

A cceptance is the path to making peace with ourselves and others.

U nderstanding ourselves gives us clarity and wisdom to know what we want, and importantly, what we don't.

T rust attunes our heart and mind so we can nurture spontaneity and adventure in our lives, and see that…

Y ou have what it takes to create the life and love you know you deserve and to never settle for anything less.

As you read this book and start to incorporate the techniques into your daily life you will see clearly that our faces tell the story of our feelings. Looking good is about feeling good and maintaining healthy skin inside and out is a big part of that.

Learning to understand the connection between how we look after our faces and how we think (stress) helps us discover our own path to an energised, vibrant and healthful face.

For when we let go of the stressful thoughts and feelings, we give ourselves a natural face lift; as self belief will out-do, out perform and outlast plastic surgery, botox, and restylane face fillers every time.

We cultivate beauty by remembering our humanness, our goodness and celebrating the best in ourselves and others

GREGORY LANDSMAN

IT'S NOT WRINKLES THAT CHANGE THE SHAPE OF THE FACE WITH AGE, BUT SAGGING MUSCLES & SKIN!

WHY FACE FITNESS AND A NATURAL LIFT WORKS!

Every major muscle on the face can be shaped and strengthened. And like any other muscle in the body, if muscles are not exercised, they will become weak and begin to sag. **Face Fitness** techniques strengthen the muscles, supporting the skin to be tight and toned while reducing and softening wrinkles. A truly healthy preventative against skin aging.

WHY FACE FITNESS LASTS LONGER THAN ANY FACE LIFT

Unlike the rest of the body where muscles are attached to bones, facial muscles are attached directly to the skin. This means that as the muscles weaken, skin sags and the face drops.

Face lifts are designed to tighten the skin by disconnecting the muscle from the skin and then pulling and stitching the muscles higher on the face. The trouble is that because a muscle isn't exercised, even after it has been surgically pulled, it will eventually sag once again. It simply has to; as the only long term solution we have to fight gravity on our faces or our bodies is exercise!

So regardless of your age, your level of stress or whether you have had a face lift or not, **Face Fitness** will help you regain and retain strong facial muscles that will support the skin to stay firm and healthy. All it takes is 10 minutes a day.

HOW FACE FITNESS WORKS

Facial muscles can be made strong and vital, restoring facial tone through detoxifying the skin (from the impacts of the environment; pollution, diet, artificial heat and air conditioning), de-stressing the face and strengthening the facial muscle framework, which results in firmer skin and the smoothing out of wrinkles.

10 MINUTES TO A NEW FACE!

It takes ten minutes per day to do the **Face Fitness** routine to support and uplift the muscles of your face, while energising, oxygenating and de-stressing the face. This time-effective, results driven routine can take 10 years off your face.

FACIAL REJUVENATING MOVEMENTS DO AMAZING THINGS!

The **Face Fitness** routine works on different levels. The daily tension we feel in our lives restricts blood vessels causing slower circulation to the facial tissues, which reduces the amount of oxygen and nutrients being received. The cumulative effect is often **pursed lips, frown lines and sagging skin**. The following techniques help you see an improvement in each of these areas.

Circulation: The routine **increases blood circulation** by freeing constrictions in the facial muscles and in the connective tissue giving the facial muscles a lift as the increased blood flow assists in bringing nutrition to the skin and removing toxins.

Skin: Elastin and collagen form the structure of our skin, but as we age we lose elasticity. The elasticity and health of our skin is determined by the tone and strength of the underlying facial muscles. **Face Fitness** helps tone and promote suppleness by stimulating muscle fibres and loosening dead skin cells, exposing fresher younger skin.

Energy: There are energy centres and meridian lines all over the body. **Face Fitness** helps to balance the energy levels on the facial pressure points, release energy blocks and bring fresh energy to the face.

Nervous system: Touch has a direct impact on emotion; **Face Fitness** can calm the nervous system, aid relaxation and reduce stress.

THE FACE FITNESS ROUTINE
ensures your face looks the best it can for as long as it can.

To be true to your beauty

You must be true to your heart

From this day forward

Never excuse who you are

Reach out

Touch life with your body

Embrace life with your mind

Remember beauty with your thoughts

Feel it with your heart

Start to live it

Beauty is your birth right

Claim it.

CONTENTS

FACE FITNESS ROUTINE PART 1 — 12
MUSCLE REVIVER MOVEMENTS — 14

FACE FITNESS ROUTINE PART 2 — 20
MUSCLE STRENGTHENING CONTRACTIONS AND ACTIONS — 22
RUB OUT THE WRINKLE — 34
AIR CARE — 35

FACE FITNESS ROUTINE PART 3 — 37
5 DAY SKIN FIRMING DIET RECIPES — 38

FACE FITNESS ROUTINE PART 4 — 45
SUPPORTING FACE UP — 46
FACE UP DAILY PLANNER — 48
FACE FOOD — 50
THE GOOD LIVING FORMULA — 56

PART 1
FACE FITNESS MASSAGE

In order for true beauty to transform our lives, faith and self-belief must also be present

In the world of fashion I have worked with faces right around the world and realised that no amount of make up, lighting or air brushing can hide a face full of stress. Stress has become our face's constant companion and is unfortunately one of the major causes for premature aging.

In today's world we carry stress in our bodies and visibly on our faces. In fact our faces say it all; how much sleep we have had; how much alcohol we have consumed, how many glasses of water we haven't or how we are feeling.

We all have different ways of dealing with stress; some run, hit the gym or swim – anything to alleviate the tension. Yet while we are busy eliminating the stress from the muscles in our body, we often neglect the fifty-seven muscles in our face.

We seem to take it for granted that we can smile, sneeze, laugh, yawn and express our feelings with our faces, but we pay little or no attention to the facial muscles that make this possible.

So while many of us are givers; to our children, our partners, our homes and our friends, it is easy to forget to give to ourselves. **Face Fitness** is about ensuring we make time to give something of real value to ourselves.

RELEASING STRESS FROM THE FACIAL MUSCLES

Massage speeds up lymphatic drainage which removes toxins and de-stresses the muscles on the face and neck that cause crow's feet, wrinkled lips, a sagging jawline, heavy jowls and frown lines.

Things you need to know...

This routine can be done first thing in the morning or last thing at night before the contraction movements.

Before you start, rub hands together vigorously and place over the face to energise.

Oil is required to provide a thin surface for hands to glide over, so the skin is not pulled or stretched.

With all of the reviver movements, work upwards. This way the veins benefit most from the blood circulation created through this process.

Start with a slow speed and increase the speed as you go, ensuring that the skin has only slight pressure placed on it.

Be aware that as you do the exercises your skin may appear red or slightly blotchy immediately afterwards. This simply shows that it is working and that there is additional circulation in the area.

As you go through the routine, notice that when you have negative thoughts, they affect your breathing, bringing on shallow breaths that weaken emotional and physical health. Breathe deeply and slowly and you will feel your facial muscles relax. Let each breath empower you and let go of the stress and tension.

FACE FITNESS REVIVER 1

When we begin to celebrate more of who we are and criticise ourselves less, our true beauty is revealed to us

DESTRESSING JOWLS

Using flat palms and moving upwards one at a time, massage the muscle of the cheek in a circular, rolling motion.

Afterwards rub hands together until hot and place over the jowls.

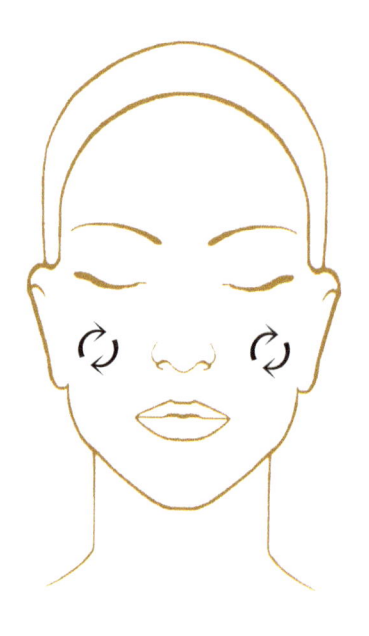

WHY IT WORKS:
Stimulates blood circulation and nourishes the tissues by carrying oxygen, which is essential to cell growth and helps to drain excess fluids in the tissue to reduce sagging.

FACE FITNESS REVIVER 2

Expressing gratitude for who you are not only boosts self esteem but nourishes your soul

DESTRESSING WRINKLED LIPS

Stretch the lips tightly by smiling; then start at the edge of the corners of the mouth and massage in circular movements from the corners to the middle, along the edge of the top lip. Swap hands and repeat on the lower lip.

Afterwards rub hands together until hot and place over the lips.

WHY IT WORKS:
Strengthens, nourishes and tones muscle fibres and clears away surface dead skin cells.

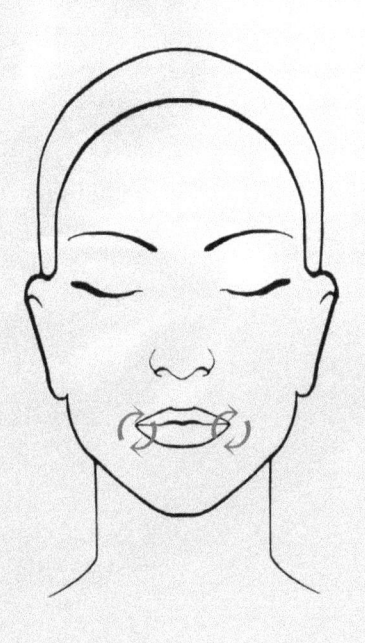

FACE FITNESS REVIVER 3

When we change how we think about ourselves from the negative to the positive, healing and self growth can take place

DESTRESSING FROWN AND BROW LINES

Using three fingers rub the forehead upwards from the brows to the hairline in a continuous movement – using one hand and then the other.

Afterwards rub hands together until hot and place over the forehead.

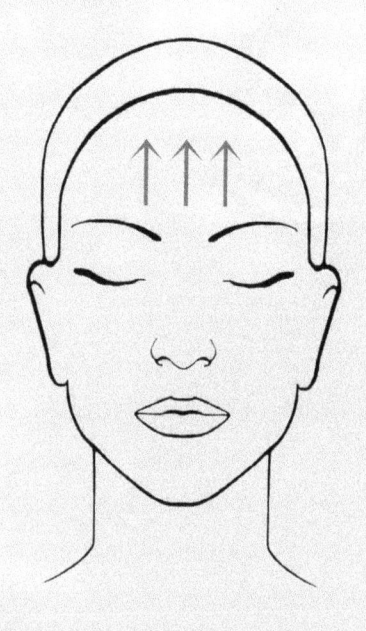

WHY IT WORKS: Maintains the moisture content of the cells supporting the skin's texture to remain dewy by stimulating the production of sebum.

FACE FITNESS REVIVER 4

Beauty is experienced through our feelings and nurtured with our thoughts

DESTRESSING CROW'S FEET

Take the middle finger on each hand and place in a crossroads position where crow's feet are emerging on one eye at a time. Use alternate middle fingers to massage out from the corner of your eye and up towards the temple.

Afterwards rub hands together until hot and place over the eye area.

WHY IT WORKS: Helps to drain excess fluids in the facial tissues, reducing sagging areas while toning and nourishing the whole area.

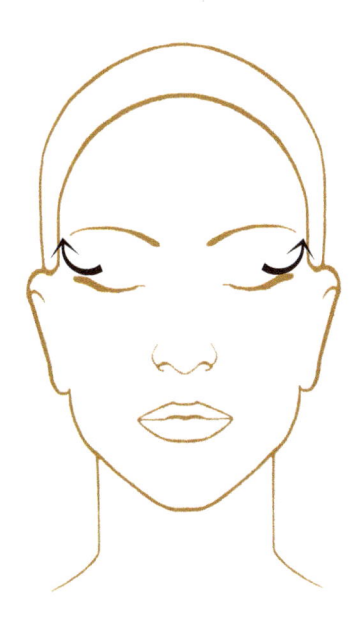

FACE FITNESS REVIVER 5

Your face can paint a thousand words
but your heart tells the story

DESTRESSING NECK AND JAWLINE

Working from the bottom of the neck to the jawline from ear to ear use both hands alternately, sliding up the neck, and working lightly over the wind pipe.

Then take the first and middle fingers of each hand and with one above and one below the jaw, massage along the jawline from the chin to ear working outwards.

Afterwards rub hands together until hot and place over the neck area.

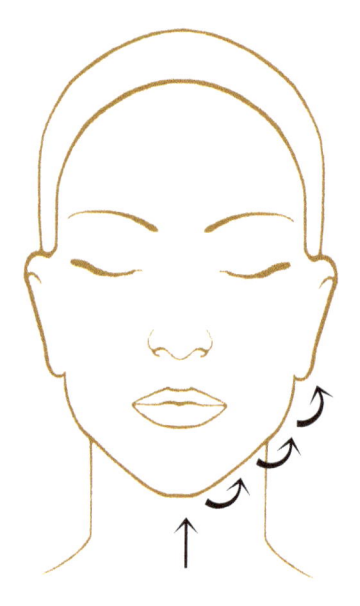

WHY IT WORKS: Fat cells in the subcutaneous tissue are minimised, strengthening the muscle fibres and firming the skin.

Every breath you take is so simple
and miraculous. So fine, it is invisible.
So intricate, it is difficult to comprehend.
Yet the simple act of breathing brings
the power of life.

Our breath is a wonderful reminder
of the beauty we are given. It is so much a
part of our daily existence that more often
than not we forget it is even there.

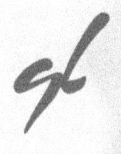

PART 2

FACE FITNESS FACIAL MUSCLE CONTRACTIONS AND ACTIONS

You are as young as your self belief, as wise as your words, as old as your doubts and as beautiful as the love you hold in your heart

TIME TO START

So now that you are aware of the muscles in your face, it is time for contraction and action! These movements are fast and easy, and will take no longer than six minutes – less once you become familiar with them. Do them at least once per day, twice for even better results.

To start you don't need any tools. Keep in mind that some of the muscles on your face have probably never been exercised before. Just breathe, relax and make sure you are in a comfortable position as you do each exercise.

The contraction exercises can be done as a routine or randomly throughout the day (in any order) – at the traffic lights, while drying your hair, watching TV or in the shower.

Also remember to start gently and be patient with yourself. Because you have probably never moved the muscles on the face in this way they will take a little time to respond.

But if you keep at it you will very quickly see the muscles start to respond, and the results that come from regular application.

When doing the contraction exercises, work the muscles to the point where you feel them burn slightly, using your fingers as weights to provide resistance. Muscles grow bigger and stronger and work harder as a result.

Another thing to keep in mind is to breathe deeply and feel the energy that is flowing through your facial muscles as you do the actions. Try not to be distracted and focus only on the muscles being contracted.

While we pay attention to the muscles on our body it is important to pay equal attention to the facial and neck muscles. Exercising the muscles will increase their strength, elasticity and size, which will ultimately plump up the skin on the face and neck.

Face Fitness will strengthen:

- The muscles around the eyes
- The cheek muscles
- The muscles that surround the mouth
- The chin muscles
- The neck muscles
- The muscles on the head and forehead
- The jaw muscles

As muscle fibres are strengthened, built and toned, they are also shortened. This will bring a more defined jawline, lifted jowls, higher cheek bones, more open eyes and higher eyebrows. As muscle fibre builds it pushes out fine lines and deeper wrinkles, revealing smoother, tighter, fresher looking skin.

FACE FITNESS

CONTRACTION 1
REDUCE EYE WRINKLES

Your beauty is the highest reflection of your thoughts and beliefs.
When you change the beliefs about your beauty, your beauty changes as well

This action aims at reducing wrinkles around the eyes while tightening and toning the entire eye area. It strengthens the muscle that is responsible for opening and closing the eye by pumping blood into the area and firming the upper and lower eyelids that begin to sag. It also plumps out and lifts under eye hollows.

Place your middle and index fingers either side of your eyes in a 'V' shape with the ends sitting just under the brow bone at both ends. Squint strongly and release 20 times then hold the squint, while pulling your eyes shut tightly and count to 30. You will feel the outer muscle of the eye pulsing.

The key is to hold your eyes closed and tight while counting to 30.

FACE FITNESS

TIP: *Make sure that you hold the skin firmly so that it doesn't move when you contract the muscle. This way it doesn't stress the skin around the eyes. Do the eye exercise twice a day to correct under eye puffiness and deep under eye hollows.*

WHY IT WORKS: With every contraction old damaged cells are cleared away leaving the skin healthier and increasing the skin's ability to absorb moisture. As the muscle fibres build, strengthen and become toned, the skin tightens around them pushing out, smoothing and flattening wrinkles.

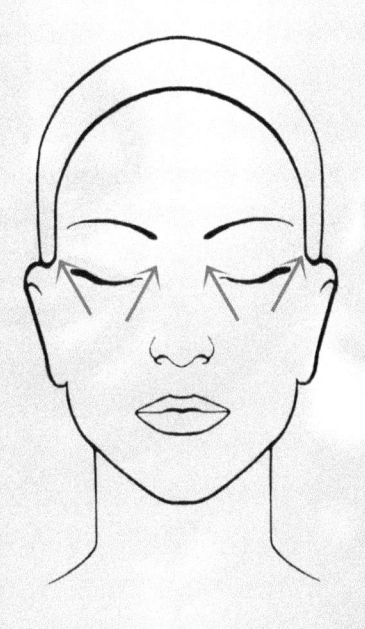

FACE FITNESS

CONTRACTION 2
ELIMINATE FROWN LINES

Beauty and ugliness exist in all of us and which one we feel depends on the thoughts we have and decisions we make day-by-day, hour-by-hour, moment-by-moment.

This action works to eliminate frown lines by working the muscles that raise the eyebrows and move the scalp forward and backwards. The forehead push up prevents and reduces frown lines and also works at counteracting heavy hooded upper eyelids.

Place two fingers from each hand on the forehead above the brows. Press fingers down and simultaneously raise the eyebrows up and down 20 times. You will feel the pressure across the forehead. Then hold the eyebrows up with the fingers still pressing down and count to 30. Then release.

FACE FITNESS

TIP: Keep the finger taut and do this exercise slowly to really work the forehead muscle. Quick contractions will not be nearly as effective as slow ones. Don't forget to breathe deeply as you do these exercises. This is a great exercise to do at traffic lights.

WHY IT WORKS: The contraction tones and smoothes the underlying muscle, the skin lifts and lines become less intense. Contracting facial muscles delivers a result 8 times greater than if you did nothing. Every contraction stimulates collagen and elastin production, which gives the skin elasticity and strength.

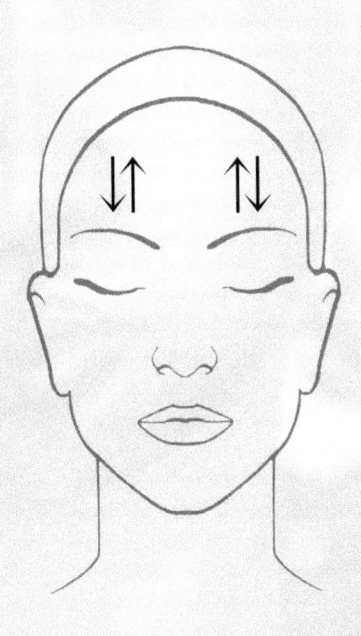

FACE FITNESS

CONTRACTION 3
ENHANCE CHEEK BONES AND CREATE YOUTHFUL CHEEKS

You do everything to look your best not because you need to impress people. You look your best because that is how you acknowledge and celebrate all aspects of who you are inside and out

As we age the cheek muscles flatten out. This action works the rounded top muscle, the apple part of the cheek and the circular muscle that surrounds the mouth. It strengthens, lifts and plumps the cheeks while simultaneously filling the under eye hollows.

Place two fingers on each cheekbone, at right angles to the face. Open the mouth and form a tight 'O' shape (squeezing the mouth muscles into the 'O' shape), then pull the lips wide while maintaining the 'O' (the upper lip must be pressing against the teeth). Squeeze the cheek muscles upwards tightly and release 30 times – this can be achieved by trying to smile in this position.

Push the muscle up under your cheek and see it moving. The two fingers on each cheek will tell you when the cheek muscle is pulsing.

FACE FITNESS

TIP: This one may feel a bit strange when you first start but over time the cheek muscles will become stronger. This exercise can be done when you are watching television.

WHY IT WORKS: Building muscle fibre enlarges the muscle and creates a natural lift, giving the cheeks a higher, more defined look. Within every square centimetre of the skin there are at least a dozen oil glands. The **Face Fitness** exercises stimulate the skin to produce natural lubricants and squeeze some of the sebum (oil) to the skin surface giving skin a natural healthy glow.

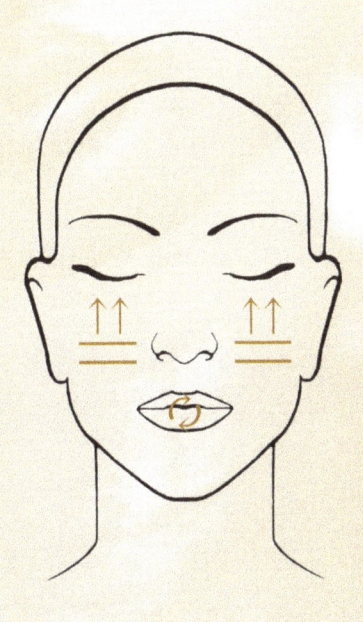

FACE FITNESS

CONTRACTION 4
ELIMINATE AND PREVENT LINES AROUND THE MOUTH

The beauty question is always what are you doing with what you have?

If your answer is 'not much' then that is what you'll get, not much.

Beauty rewards come from effort not excuses

This action strengthens the muscle around the mouth, smoothing out lines around the mouth and enlarging lips for a fuller, firmer look.

Place a finger from each hand inside the mouth and pull the mouth wide at the corners. Squeeze the muscles of the mouth to pull the fingers back together then release, taking the fingers and mouth wide once again.

Repeat 15 times.

FACE FITNESS

TIP: *This one may feel a bit strange when you first start but over time the cheek muscles will become stronger. This exercise can be done when you are watching television.*

WHY IT WORKS: Building muscle fibre enlarges the muscle and creates a natural lift, giving the cheeks a higher, more defined look. Within every square centimetre of the skin there are at least a dozen oil glands. The **Face Fitness** exercises stimulate the skin to produce natural lubricants and squeeze some of the sebum (oil) to the skin surface giving skin a natural healthy glow.

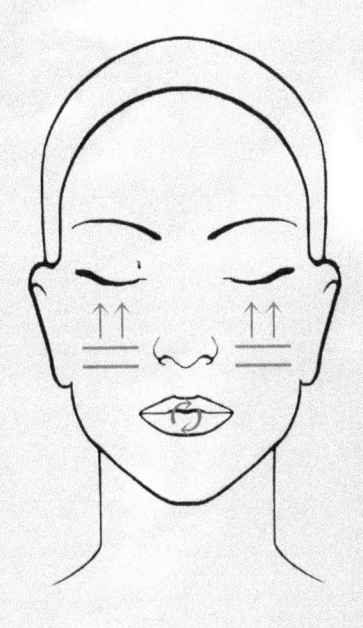

FACE FITNESS 27

FACE FITNESS

CONTRACTION 4
ELIMINATE AND PREVENT LINES AROUND THE MOUTH

The beauty question is always what are you doing with what you have?

If your answer is 'not much' then that is what you'll get, not much.

Beauty rewards come from effort not excuses

This action strengthens the muscle around the mouth, smoothing out lines around the mouth and enlarging lips for a fuller, firmer look.

Place a finger from each hand inside the mouth and pull the mouth wide at the corners. Squeeze the muscles of the mouth to pull the fingers back together then release, taking the fingers and mouth wide once again.

Repeat 15 times.

FACE FITNESS

TIP: *Don't pull too hard on the mouth when it is wide as this will stress the muscles. The stretch to be achieved here is gentle and the contraction of the mouth pulls the fingers together. Don't forget to maintain steady breathing. This is a great exercise to release tension from lips.*

WHY IT WORKS: Contracting the muscles builds fibres while simultaneously plumping the tissue. This reduces and prevents the appearance of fine lines. On average each square centimetre of skin contains approximately 1 metre of tiny blood vessels and 100 sweat glands. With every contraction the blood is oxygenated and supports the removal of toxins in the skin.

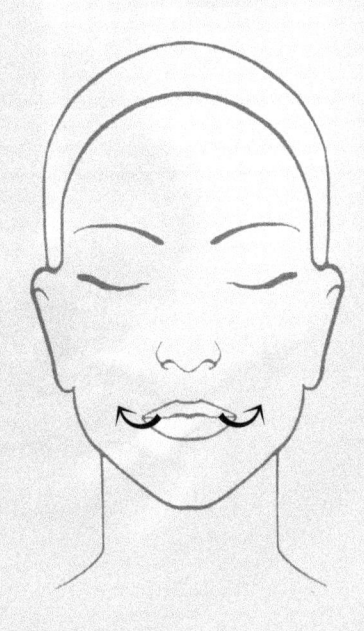

FACE FITNESS

CONTRACTION 5
REDUCE JOWLS

The ultimate expression of our willingness to feel our beauty is when we confront and conquer our fears. So when it comes to beauty, live by the two C's – confront and conquer

This action strengthens the muscle from the nose to the corner of the mouth which plumps up, reduces and prevents jowl lines.

Form a tight 'O' with the mouth, with the lips tightly pressed against the upper teeth. Pull you mouth wide with a smile (while holding the 'O' shape) and pull your nose upwards, so that you can feel it pulling on the sides of your nose and release. Repeat this 20 times and then on the final tightening hold for 20 and release.

FACE FITNESS

TIP: The muscles around the nose may not even feel like they are moving when you first start this exercise, but do it in a mirror and keep at it. Eventually you will see movement as they get stronger. You will also see results very quickly. Do these regularly and maintain steady breathing.

WHY IT WORKS: The contraction works the muscle and connective tissue increasing the strength and tone, while lifting the jowls. This plumps out the skin making it both smoother and younger looking.

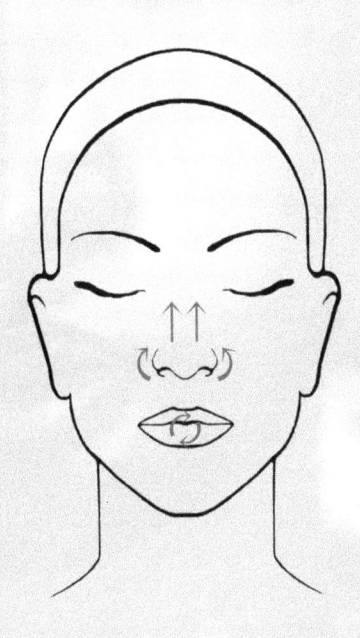

FACE FITNESS

CONTRACTION 6
TIGHTEN NECK AND JAWLINE

Feeling your beauty for just a moment is a creative self enlarging experience. It allows us to develop spontaneity and to let go of old beliefs that keep us feeling stuck

This action strengthens and firms the primary neck muscle to smooth and counteract sagging skin, while pumping up the jaw muscle to lift a sagging jawline and reduce double chins.

Push your tongue out as far as you can and smile so that the skin on the neck is sucked up under the chin. Return the tongue back into the mouth and repeat the movement 15 times. You will feel this working all the way up the neck and across the entire jaw line. On the last contraction hold and squeeze the muscles while counting to 10.

FACE FITNESS

TIP: *When pushing the tongue out do it slowly. Hold it out for the count of one and then pull it back in and repeat the movement.*

WHY IT WORKS: Skin cells thrive on exercise. The more you exercise the facial muscles, the more revitalised your skin becomes, which improves both colour and muscle tone. When muscles on the face and neck are developed they reach their optimal strength and as the muscle fibres build, the skin is lifted creating a more defined neck and jaw line.

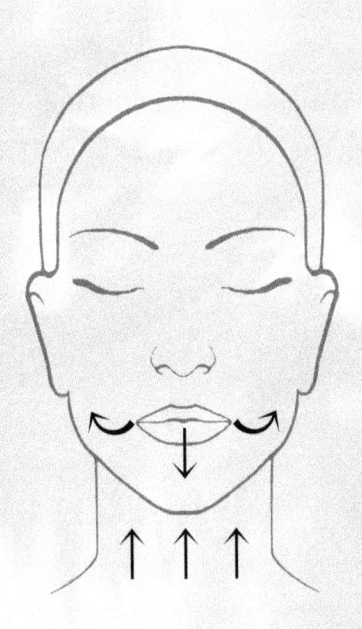

FACE FITNESS
RUB OUT THE WRINKLE

Work hard to experience beauty but never hurt yourself to find it or keep it

Ensure the skin has been cleansed then cover the area that you want to concentrate on lightly with oil or moisturiser.

Deep wrinkles are caused by skin that is tacked down to underlying tissue. This technique de-tacks the skin, rubbing out fine lines and reducing the appearance of deeper-set wrinkles.

For horizontal wrinkles work the fingers vertically, for vertical wrinkles work the fingers horizontally.

Take a finger from each hand and have them work in opposite directions to each other, moving one finger gently one way, while the other moves the opposite direction (without stretching or placing pressure on the wrinkle).

Do this up to 25 times or until you see the skin becoming red from increased blood flow.

Next, hold a finger at either side of the wrinkle (one above, one below for a horizontal wrinkle). Then take a finger from the other hand and rub out the wrinkle, rubbing your finger gently back and forth until the skin changes to deep red. Do this up to 5 or 6 times to begin with, more as you continue the treatment.

Note: once the skin becomes used to the treatment you can apply harder pressure but this must be built up gradually.

FACE FITNESS

TIGHTEN AND TONE CHEEKS, LIPS AND JOWLS

There is no such thing as perfect beauty, only human beauty...

This technique can be done anywhere and any time. Simply fill your mouth with air and hold the air bubble in. Continue to breathe through your nose. Move the air bubble around from cheek to cheek and circulate it around your mouth in a variety of directions.

This technique is simple, but delivers powerful results as it tones and gives the mid-face (cheek muscles, muscles around the mouth and chin) a gentle work out. Keep rotating the air in all directions. Start with one cheek at a time and then move the air to all the other areas, upper lips, lower lips, near the chin. Move the air clockwise and anticlockwise.

Do this for at least twenty seconds and release. Repeat three times.

This releases blocked energy and reduces tension and stress in the entire area.

Remember that as with all exercise, the first month is the hardest.
But nothing great is achieved without commitment, so keep in mind that the more you train, the more results you gain.
Train a minimum of once or twice a day depending on what you want to achieve.

The first law of true beauty is structure.
Notice how everything that grows in nature,
whether a tree or a rose, has structure.
Nature keeps what is essential and gets rid of
what is not needed for growth.
For beauty to grow we must have structure,
not bone structure but
structure with what we do to ourselves in
thought, word and deed.

PART 3
5 DAY SKIN FIRMING DIET
(NUTRITIONAL FACE LIFT)

A healthy diet is what supports your face to look healthy and vital. What we put on the inside shows up on the outside. Here are some food guidelines to keep the skin looking fresh and radiant.

Avoid Crash Diets as you lose lean muscle tissue, which causes skin to sag and the face to become drawn. Losing weight gradually allows your skin to shrink gently, so the elastin and collagen fibres can become accustomed to the change.

Fruits and vegetables - are all good but berries (such as blackberries, strawberries, blueberries and raspberries) are strong antioxidants and are great for fighting free radicals, which damage skin cells. Bright coloured vegetables are also good for the skin.

Water – we need a minimum of eight glasses of water a day to flush out and eliminate toxins and purify the body.

Green Tea – is loaded with antioxidants that reduce inflammation and fight free radicals that cause skin damage. Adding some lemon juice is twice as beneficial.

Selenium – Is a power packed nutrient found in Brazil Nuts, whole grain breads, turkey and tuna. Include one of these in your daily diet.

Dairy (Low fat) – Yoghurt (natural low fat) – has a high vitamin A content which is beneficial to the skin and aids the digestive system.

To achieve healthy glowing skin eat food rich in Omega fatty acids, minerals, Vitamin C and zinc.

To Avoid Inflammation of the Skin reduce salt and eliminate white flour, rice (choose brown or Basmati), pasta and sugar. Also eliminate processed foods as they are loaded with sugar and additives that rob the skin of essential nutrients. Sugar also causes premature aging as it blocks Vitamin C functions, which are essential for collagen and elastin production.

For best results cut out all dairy products (with the exception of low fat yoghurt) and coffee from your diet.

FIVE DAY
SKIN FIRMING DIET RECIPES

As part of my program of learning in India I was taught about the anti-aging benefits of Indian spices and how potent the combination of good diet and the right face techniques could be.

I created the five day skin firming diet to support the **Face Fitness** routine by nurturing your skin with food that is full of antioxidants and anti aging ingredients.

If you can't eat one of the recipes, substitute it with a recipe from another day. Whatever you choose, keep in mind that regular inclusions of fish will provide your diet with fish oil which is wonderful for the skin and a known anti-inflammatory.

Follow this eating program for five days and see the results. You will find your face loses excess fluid and puffiness, fine lines will be less apparent, skin will feel tighter and that the skin will start to regain its natural glow.

Adapt and incorporate the key elements into your lifestyle and continue to support your face with a nutritional face lift.

Note: There are no set amounts of most ingredients in these recipes. That is because their success doesn't rely on specific measurements, but rather the use of all ingredients in moderation. Remember, this isn't a diet for losing weight (although you might) – this regime is all about your skin. So if you would like a little extra olive oil, ginger, chilli or any other ingredient, it's up to you!

FIVE DAY SKIN FIRMING DIET RECIPES

As part of my program of learning in India I was taught about the anti-aging benefits of Indian spices and how potent the combination of good diet and the right face techniques could be.

I created the five day skin firming diet to support the **Face Fitness** routine by nurturing your skin with food that is full of antioxidants and anti aging ingredients.

If you can't eat one of the recipes, substitute it with a recipe from another day. Whatever you choose, keep in mind that regular inclusions of fish will provide your diet with fish oil which is wonderful for the skin and a known anti-inflammatory.

Follow this eating program for five days and see the results. You will find your face loses excess fluid and puffiness, fine lines will be less apparent, skin will feel tighter and that the skin will start to regain its natural glow.

Adapt and incorporate the key elements into your lifestyle and continue to support your face with a nutritional face lift.

Note: There are no set amounts of most ingredients in these recipes. That is because their success doesn't rely on specific measurements, but rather the use of all ingredients in moderation. Remember, this isn't a diet for losing weight (although you might) – this regime is all about your skin. So if you would like a little extra olive oil, ginger, chilli or any other ingredient, it's up to you!

PART 3
5 DAY SKIN FIRMING DIET
(NUTRITIONAL FACE LIFT)

A healthy diet is what supports your face to look healthy and vital. What we put on the inside shows up on the outside. Here are some food guidelines to keep the skin looking fresh and radiant.

Avoid Crash Diets as you lose lean muscle tissue, which causes skin to sag and the face to become drawn. Losing weight gradually allows your skin to shrink gently, so the elastin and collagen fibres can become accustomed to the change.

Fruits and vegetables - are all good but berries (such as blackberries, strawberries, blueberries and raspberries) are strong antioxidants and are great for fighting free radicals, which damage skin cells. Bright coloured vegetables are also good for the skin.

Water – we need a minimum of eight glasses of water a day to flush out and eliminate toxins and purify the body.

Green Tea – is loaded with antioxidants that reduce inflammation and fight free radicals that cause skin damage. Adding some lemon juice is twice as beneficial.

Selenium – Is a power packed nutrient found in Brazil Nuts, whole grain breads, turkey and tuna. Include one of these in your daily diet.

Dairy (Low fat) – Yoghurt (natural low fat) – has a high vitamin A content which is beneficial to the skin and aids the digestive system.

To achieve healthy glowing skin eat food rich in Omega fatty acids, minerals, Vitamin C and zinc.

To Avoid Inflammation of the Skin reduce salt and eliminate white flour, rice (choose brown or Basmati), pasta and sugar. Also eliminate processed foods as they are loaded with sugar and additives that rob the skin of essential nutrients. Sugar also causes premature aging as it blocks Vitamin C functions, which are essential for collagen and elastin production.

For best results cut out all dairy products (with the exception of low fat yoghurt) and coffee from your diet.

FACE FITNESS

MONDAY

BREAKFAST
1 cup of boiled water with half a fresh lemon squeezed into it.
1 egg white omelette (3 egg whites) and a pinch of cumin,
do not add salt.
1 serve of fruit.
1-2 glasses of water.

LUNCH
1 small can of tuna mixed with 1 chopped tomato, half a cucumber and a handful of spinach leaves, topped with walnuts.
Squeeze half a fresh lemon and a teaspoon of olive oil over the salad.
Optional: add some cumin and chilli to the salad dressing.
Green tea and two glasses of water.

DINNER
Grilled chicken fillet with a mixed salad.
Green tea and two glasses of water.
Optional: make a mixture of curry powder, cumin, ginger, garlic and a tablespoon of olive oil as a paste for coating the chicken.

SNACK
Pears, cantaloupe, almonds.

Berry smoothie:
¾ cup of strawberries
¾ cup of blackberries
½ cup of plain low fat yoghurt
1 cup of crushed ice

This drink is loaded with Vitamins A, B1, B6 and folic acid, which aids in the formation of healthy cell formation. Adding fresh berries protects skin from free radicals and helps maintain healthy capillaries.

Lemon Water is not only cleansing to the body, it contains Vitamin C which assists in collagen production and the elasticity (firmness) of the skin.

TUESDAY

BREAKFAST
1 cup of boiled water with half a fresh lemon squeezed into it.
1 cup of non fat yoghurt with some strawberries and an apple or pear chopped up and mixed in.
1-2 glasses of water.

LUNCH
1 tin of small sardines with tomato, cucumber and lettuce, finished with fresh lemon juice.
Optional: add chilli or cumin to the lemon dressing.
1 serve of fruit.
2 glasses of lemon water.

DINNER
Skinless chicken roasted with mushrooms, 1 zucchini and four cloves of garlic served on a bed of spinach. Season with fresh lemon juice, a teaspoon of virgin olive oil, ginger and fresh mint.
1 cup of hot lemon water.

SNACK
Pineapple Orange Juice:
1 cup fresh pineapple
½ an orange
½ a lime

This juice is loaded with minerals that are great skin boosters; Magnesium, calcium, sodium, phosphorous, iron and iodine. It is also rich in Vitamins C, A and B complex.

Strawberries are part of the berry family, which has some of the highest total antioxidant capacity of any food. Antioxidants fight free radicals and assist in protecting the skin from premature aging.

Garlic is not only known as a 'blood cleanser' but is high in Sulphur which helps smooth the surface of the skin.

WEDNESDAY

BREAKFAST
1 cup of hot lemon water.
1 cup of unflavoured oatmeal with a sliced pear.
1-2 glasses of lemon water.

LUNCH
1 small tin of salmon on parsley, lettuce and tomato salad, dressed with 1 teaspoon of lemon juice and olive oil.
Optional: add chilli, cumin and turmeric to the salad dressing.
1 piece of melon, an apple or a pear.
2 glasses of lemon water.

DINNER
Sautéed chicken strips with assorted vegetables - zucchini, broccoli and cauliflower. Season with fresh herbs, a teaspoon of olive oil and lemon, a pinch of cumin and some black pepper.
1 cup of hot lemon water.

Remember to drink a minimum of eight glasses of water including the lemon water.

SNACK
Apple beet juice:
Process ½ a large beet and two apples in a juicer.

This nutritional punch is quite strong and can be diluted with water. It is loaded with calcium, sulphur, potassium and iron which are essential for healthy red blood cells.

Oatmeal contains Vitamin E, a powerful antioxidant and Zinc which is essential for building healthy skin.

Melon replenishes the skin's antioxidant levels helping to protect the skin while counteracting dryness.

Beets are a power skin food containing Vitamins A and C, phosphorous, calcium and magnesium, which are skin renewing and skin building.

Cumin seeds are full of Vitamin E, an antioxidant which helps heal skin tissue and keep it healthy and glowing.

THURSDAY

BREAKFAST
1 cup of hot lemon water.
1 egg white omelette with spinach.
1 piece of fresh fruit.
1-2 glasses of lemon water.

LUNCH
1 small tin of tuna or sardines and half a cup of bean salad.
Optional: add a little curry powder, chilli and/or ginger to the bean salad.
1 piece of fresh fruit.
2 glasses of lemon water.

DINNER
Chicken done with lemon juice, honey, ginger and fresh coriander served with asparagus, bean sprouts, garlic and zucchini.
2 glasses of lemon water before bed.

SNACK
Green Juice:
2 green apples
2 cups of spinach
½ a cup of parsley

Process ingredients together in a juicer. This juice is loaded with Vitamins A and C, iron and the antioxidant lutein.

Oily Fish is full of essential fatty acids that are responsible for healthy cell membranes that protect the moisture levels in the skin, which ensures plumper healthier looking skin. Eating salmon at least three times per week will reduce puffiness on the face and support firmness.

Egg whites contain magnesium, potassium and selenium which are all skin building essential minerals.

Green vegetables are full of Vitamin A which support cell turnover. Without Vitamin A, skin can become dry and scaly.

Ginger is known to be good for digestion and calming the stomach, but it is also an anti-inflammatory.

FRIDAY

BREAKFAST
1 cup of hot lemon water.
Salmon egg white omelette (3 egg whites) seasoned with fresh parsley and a pinch of cumin.
1 piece of fresh fruit.
1-2 glasses of lemon water.

LUNCH
Steamed vegetables with 1 fillet of skinless grilled chicken, seasoned with fresh basil, lemon juice and virgin olive oil.
Optional: add chilli and garlic mixed with a tablespoon of olive oil and baste the chicken while grilling.
1 piece of fresh fruit.
2 glasses of lemon water.

DINNER
Pan fried chicken fillet or salmon, 1 small tin tomatoes with chopped capsicum, zucchini, onion and a clove of garlic. Season with lemon juice, olive oil and fresh herbs of your choice.
1 piece of fresh fruit.
2 glasses of lemon water.

SNACK
Orange Refresher:
2 oranges
1 apple
½ a cup of ice

Process ingredients in a blender. This drink is loaded with Vitamin C which aids in building collagen.

Salmon contains Vitamins A and D, essential minerals zinc, calcium and selenium, and Omega-3 fatty acids – a power packed skin boosting food.

Parsley contains high levels of Vitamin C, iron and potassium which together build collagen and strengthen the connective tissue of skin.

Capsicum contains Vitamins A and C, essential for the renewing and growth of skin, and also holds anti-inflammatory properties.

There will always be times when you will feel challenged by the world's concept of beauty. Times when you will feel that deeply cherished thoughts about what you thought made you valuable must be left behind, so that you choose to believe in the truth of who you are and find it in yourself once again.

This is the time to create a new vision of ourselves.

Let this vision be born from the wisdom of knowing our beauty as human beings.

PART 4

10 THINGS THAT STRESS AND AGE OUR BODIES AND SHOW UP ON OUR FACES...

While genetic factors play a major role in the way we age, so does lifestyle.

In our health conscious society, the words, "You look stressed," are very familiar. If we are not saying them to ourselves, we are saying them to others.

Here are 10 things (in no particular order) that contribute to aging and stress being stored in our bodies and showing up on our faces.

1. EXCESS ALCOHOL
2. MENTAL ANXIETY
3. SMOKING AND DRUGS
4. LOW EXERCISE
5. SATURATED FATS
6. UNPROTECTED OR EXCESSIVE SUN EXPOSURE
7. POLLUTED AIR
8. NOT ENOUGH SLEEP
9. EXCESS WEIGHT
10. SUGAR CONSUMPTION

SUPPORTING FACE FITNESS

*When a person is self accepting,
healthy and vital, beauty arises naturally*

SLEEP
One of the quickest and most efficient ways to nourish not only your skin, but your body involves getting at least seven hours sleep. This rejuvenates the whole body. You will feel stronger and your skin will look fresher.

EXERCISE
Exercising regularly gives us an increased dose of oxygen, essential for a healthy body and to keep skin glowing. The natural glow you get after a bit of exercise comes as a result of increased blood circulation, which carries nutrients to maintain and repair skin cells and help process toxins that damage the skin. Try to exercise within your body's capability for 30 minutes per day or at least three times per week. Avoid running, as pounding the pavement pulls on the elastic fibres of the skin. Walking, swimming and cycling are preferable.

BREATHE DEEPLY
Deep breathing is a very effective way to increase your energy levels and keep your skin healthy. Become conscious of your breath. Most of us breathe using our upper lungs. Deep breathing uses our diaphragm and our lower lungs. Practise sitting up straight. Relax the shoulders. Inhale deeply through your nose, slowly filling your lungs as you breathe. When you can't breathe any more air into your lungs, hold your breath briefly and then exhale through your mouth. Do this for 10 minutes per day.

SKIN DEEP
We know that nutrients nourish the skin from the inside, but what you do on the outside also has a direct impact on your skin.

Exfoliate

Exfoliate your skin regularly to remove the dead skin cells that have been exposed to pollution and other environmental impacts.

Glycolic acid is a great exfloliator and skin rejuvenator. One of the purest forms of glycolic acid is pure castor sugar, which can be used on your face or any part of the body.

Dampen your face and gently rub the sugar in circular motions, avoiding the eye area. Leave it on for a couple of minutes and then rinse. This will help keep skin fresh and hydrated.

Cleanse, Tone and Nourish Skin

Ensure you cleanse and tone to open and clean the pores.

After cleansing in the morning use a day moisturiser. At night use a night treatment that will nourish, strengthen and rebuild your skin while you sleep.

Eye creams are unnecessary if you are using a good quality night cream.

Give yourself a mask at least once a week, as they draw out impurities from the pores while tightening and toning the skin.

A great natural mask is 1 teaspoon of yoghurt, 1 egg white and 1 teaspoon of fresh lemon juice. The alpha hydroxy acid in the yoghurt removes dead skin cells and combined with the vitamin A and B5, works as a gentle exfoliant, increasing the moisture content of the skin. The egg white tightens and tones and the Vitamin C in the lemon juice stimulates elastin and collagen production.

Relax the Face

If you feel that your face is uptight and stressed, take some Epsom salts and gently rub over the face with water. The magnesium in Epsom Salts will relax the facial muscles and help to relieve tension. This is a good weekly treatment.

FACE FITNESS DAILY PLANNER

Start every day with an intention to feel beautiful and happy. Some days will be better than others, but if beauty is your intention you will get better and better at experiencing it

Keeping a tally of how you are going on the **Face Fitness** Routine not only helps keep your approach disciplined, but builds a sense of achievement as you see clearly on the page what you have accomplished.

- Mark in the number of exercises you have done for the day for each of the Revivers and Contractions.
- Tick off the meals you ate from the 5 Day Skin Firming Diet (those that didn't include any other foods that inflame the skin.)
- Mark up the amount of water and green tea drunk for the day.
- Note the amount of sleep you've had each night, how often you are exercising and whether you are doing the breathing exercises.
- Finally, tick off whether you have looked after your skin from the outside in on a daily and weekly basis.

At the end of each week you will be able to identify any gaps and begin to understand what works for your face and what doesn't.

I recommend using this grid for at least four weeks (make up your own, mark it in pencil or photocopy it) so that you can monitor your activity and detail your success.

Undoubtedly if you get 8 hours sleep each night, stick to the diet and keep to the **Face Fitness** routine, within a very short period of time you will see a significant difference in the tone and texture of your face.

FACE FITNESS Routine	MON	TUES	WED	THURS	FRI
REVIVERS 1 Jowls 2 Lips 3 Brow Lines 4 Crow's feet 5 Jawline					
CONTRACTIONS 1 Eye Reviver 2 Forehead 3 Cheeks 4 Lips 5 Jowls 6 Neck & Jaw					
5 DAY SKIN FIRMING DIET • Breakfast • Lunch • Dinner • Snacks 8 Glasses of water Green Tea (no coffee) No added salt No dairy (except low fat yoghurt) No white flour products					
SUPPORT for FACE FITNESS Sleep (hrs) Exercise (30 mins) Breathe					
SKIN CARE Exfoliate Cleanse, Tone & Nourish Relax the face					

FACE FOOD

*When beauty is accompanied by kindness
we experience the power of our humanity*

Remember that applying food topically in the form of skin treatments is a great way to absorb nutrients and nurture your skin.

Aloe Vera
Is moisturising and soothing to the skin and regenerates healthy skin cells. It contains Vitamins C, A, E and B and a series of minerals, enzymes and amino acids which are known to be anti-inflammatory.

Apple cider vinegar
Apple cider vinegar keeps skin supple. It's heavy concentration of enzymes help peel off dead skin cells. Use as an astringent on oily skin.

Avocado
The oil in avocado tightens the skin and penetrates the layers to the deepest level. It is good for reducing fine lines and enhancing overall skin tone. Avocado contains more than 25 essential nutrients and Vitamins including high levels of Vitamins E and C, which stimulate collagen production.

Baking Soda
Baking soda is a natural exfoliant, neutraliser and skin soother.

Banana
The antioxidants and nutrients in bananas help to restore collagen in the skin. They also have antibacterial properties and can be applied to the face mashed with lemon (stops the banana going brown) or with yoghurt, honey, egg or milk for a range of benefits that assist in maintaining the health of the skin.

Barley
Barley is full of antioxidants and enzymes together with Vitamins A, B, C and E. It helps elasticity in the skin and is both regenerative and moisturising.

Carrots
Carrots are an excellent source of Vitamin A which is essential in the maintenance of healthy skin and hair, as well as Coenzyme Q10 (also found in many high quality face creams).

Citrus Fruit
Citrus fruits contain Vitamin C (collagen building) which helps neutralise free radical activity and most importantly promote collagen synthesis – the key to skin remaining youthful and elastic.

Cucumber
Cucumber contains Vitamins A and C (collagen building) and is a strong antioxidant with a number of trace minerals and enzymes essential for skin growth and repair. It is a good source of silica, a trace mineral that contributes to the strength of connective tissue. Cucumber is immediately effective on puffy eyes, sunburn or as a tonic for the whole face.

Eggs
Eggs contain Vitamins A, B5 and D, and proteins that when applied to the face have a tightening and constricting effect on the pores. When egg whites are used as a mask they also remove dead skin cells.

Epsom Salts
Epsom salts or Magnesium Sulphate is a long time remedy that has a multitude of benefits when applied topically or used for soaking.

Epsom salts have a high magnesium content and as such is a natural muscle relaxant that can assist in lowering blood pressure, reducing stress, improving sleep and calming the nervous system. In a bath the salts draw toxins through the water and absorb the nutrients through the skin. Epsom Salts are associated with helping back pain and aching limbs and also treating cold and congestion through the release of toxins.

Grapes
Grapes are high in Alpha Hydroxy Acid (AHA) which is skin renewing, and Vitamin C which is collagen building, so they are powerful for use as a skin exfoliant, for oil reduction and skin bleaching.

Honey
Honey both attracts and retains moisture and is soothing and nourishing to the skin. It contains a natural exfoliant and is hydrating and calming to sore or irritated skin. Honey can be used for all over body nourishment in a range of treatments.

Lemon
Lemons are rich in AHA and Vitamin C (collagen building) and a range of nutrients that has ensured its use as a rejuvenating beauty product for hundreds of years. Its versatility as a topical ingredient means it can be used in cleansers, toners, skin lighteners, face masks and scrubs. It is naturally antiseptic and has been used successfully to treat fine lines, scars and pigmentation of every kind.

Milk
Milk and yoghurt soften and soothe the skin because of the presence of lactic acid (AHA), a gentle exfoliant which renews and hydrates skin. High in Vitamins A and D, milk nourishes and soothes dry, itchy and irritated skin, holding natural properties that calm irritation and reduce redness.

Oatmeal
Oatmeal is appropriate for dry and sensitive skin acting as both an exfoliator and moisturiser.

Olive Oil
Olive oil is extremely high in Vitamin E and Vitamin K (found in green leafy vegetables), and contains high antioxidant and anti-inflammatory properties that help counteract exposure to pollution, smoke and alcohol. Olive oil is so rich in its nutrient value that it can be used topically on any part of the body to moisturise and regenerate.

Orange
Oranges are high in Vitamins A and C (collagen building) and are of great benefit to all skin types because of their regenerative skin properties. Oranges stimulate circulation and the release of toxins from the skin.

Papaya
Papaya is high in AHA which removes the top layer of dead cells and helps regenerate fresh new skin. It also contains Vitamins C (collagen building), E and K which support overall skin health.

Peach
Peach is a great source of antioxidants which help protect the skin from UV rays. Research has shown that nutrients from topically applied juice benefit the strength and elasticity of skin.

Pineapple
Pineapple is a citrus fruit (Vitamin C – collagen building) which contains high levels of AHA, has a hydrating effect on the skin and is also anti-inflammatory, meaning the overall result is one that promotes clearer looking skin.

Potato
Potatoes contain Vitamins C (collagen building) and B and minerals such as potassium, magnesium, phosphorus and zinc – all of which are good for the skin. Potato juice is excellent in skin packs and can assist in curing pimples and spots on the skin. It can also provide immediate relief from burns if placed directly on the area. Potatoes are also a skin cleanser and natural skin lightener.

Rose Water
Rose Water stimulates skin, balances pH levels, tightens pores and increases blood flow. It is antibacterial and appropriate for dry and oily skin.

Sugar
Sugar contains glycolic acid and is part of the AHA family, which helps break down dead skin cells leaving skin renewed and revitalised. Sugar can be applied topically to the face or the whole body as a scrub which hydrates skin without clogging pores. It can also be used as a one minute manicure or pedicure.

Sunflower Oil
Sunflower oil is a superb source of nutrients for the skin, containing Vitamins A, D and E. Vitamin E is known for its anti-inflammatory and antioxidant properties and is often used to heal scar tissue and fine lines on the face.

Tea
When applied topically the tannins in tea reduce inflammation. Tea is known for putting oxygen into the skin and fighting free radicals that are destructive.

Tomatoes
Tomatoes are rich in Vitamin A, Vitamin C (collagen building) and potassium: essential for fresh glowing skin.

Turmeric
Turmeric is a natural antibiotic, a strong antioxidant and anti-inflammatory, and acknowledged as a potent anti-aging treatment.

Vegetable Oils
Oils such as Apricot Kernel, Avocado, Almond, Peach Kernel, Jojoba, Sunflower, Sesame, Olive or Soybean are all rich in unsaturated Fatty Acids, Vitamins and minerals that are essential to maintenance of moisture levels in the skin.

Vinegar
Vinegar can help restore the natural pH balance in your skin which assists with dryness, itching and flaking. It can be used as a cleanser and toner for your skin when mixed with water.

Watermelon
Watermelon is high in the super antioxidant lycopene and Vitamins A, B and C (collagen building), which keep the skin fresh, radiant and hydrated. The natural acids act as exfoliates which are good for removing blemishes.

Yoghurt
Yoghurt contains AHA (skin renewal), Vitamins A and B5 and will act as a gentle exfoliant that increases the moisture content in skin and hair. It will also cool and soothe irritated skin.

Love has the highest vibration that
allows us to open our hearts and enlarge
the beauty in ourselves and our lives.
When we see how loveable we are
we begin to see how beautiful we are.

FACE FITNESS GOOD LIVING B.E.A.U.T.Y. RECIPES

How we live has a direct impact on how we feel and how we feel shows up on our faces. Balance, Enthusiasm, Acceptance, Understanding, Trust and You are the keys for keeping our Faces Fit.

BALANCE

Balance is not about either indulgence or repression, but in seeking balance we are encouraged to look closely at the relationships and the choices we make.

- Balance supports us to recognise that all the decisions we make ultimately shape our lives.
- Focus on exercising the muscle that people can't see – the heart.
- Breathe deeply and consciously and be mindful of the life force that flows through you.
- Do some cardiovascular exercise; it gets the heart pumping blood through the body. This gives you more endurance so you can do more without feeling lethargic.
- Practise wholeness. Eat and exercise to increase the flow of energy and nurture wholesome emotions, thoughts and acts, as they will enable you to find balance, peace and rest in yourself.
- Over indulgence in anything weakens our vitality and promotes feelings of weakness – especially self indulgence.

Keep good company with yourself and practise sitting in silence for ten minutes every day. Remember, the company you keep can help you become bigger or smaller as a person, so choose your company carefully.

ENTHUSIASM

Awakening the enthusiastic response within yourself is not about excitement, but a deep conviction that what you are and represent is a true reflection of you. The more enthusiasm we feel for ourselves, the more energy we have to participate in life and the more we can express ourselves fully.

- Develop spontaneity and let go of ideas that keep you feeling stuck and are no longer relevant. Be willing to explore new ideas that can develop your creativity and personal talents.
- Recognise beauty in the things that you do, not only in the things you have.
- Count your blessings and give up counting calories.
- Following fads dulls our consciousness, following our heart expands it.
- Never argue for your limitations only for your possibilities.
- Focus on what you have to give the world not on what the world has not given you.
- Think beauty when you look into a person's eyes, and you will begin to see it when you look into your own.
- Never forget to share a smile with a stranger, it costs nothing but brings so much.
- Play a favourite song regularly and dance in the presence of your own company.
- Develop enthusiasm as part of your character, not as a reaction to people or circumstances. Enthusiastic thoughts lead to enthusiastic feelings.

ACCEPTANCE

Self acceptance is the way we make peace with ourselves. It is not about reciting affirmations or chanting mantras, it is about making the decision to drop the judgement from our lives.

The more you accept of yourself, the more you learn to appreciate yourself. The more you recognise that the true source of feeling good about yourself and life lies within the way you think and feel, the more you are empowered to take responsibility for your own well being.

- Give up self criticism and criticism of others. Strengthen your magnetism by never making excuses for who you are or what you look like.
- Acceptance is what makes us all beautiful, so stand up for your individuality.
- Self acceptance supports our nervous system to relax and our anxieties to disappear.
- Not judging or belittling other people and respecting their differences, is what allows you to accept your own.
- Remember that the most beautiful things in life can't always be seen – the heart is one of them.
- Let no person's opinion or advertising image condition the way you see, think or feel about yourself.
- Know that acceptance comes not from changing the outside but from inner changes; thoughts, beliefs and attitudes.
- Do not restrict the way you live by the way you look. Claim inner freedom and live it.

UNDERSTANDING

Understanding ourselves gives us emotional and mental clarity, and enables us to honour who we are and the choices we make. Through understanding we begin to open up clear channels of communication with ourselves and others, which naturally opens up the way to live authentically.

- Be more concerned about what you think and feel about yourself and worry less about what others think and feel about you.
- What we have been taught about love and looks has taught us to judge ourselves from the outside in. To lead a fulfilling and happy life we need to reverse this.
- Remember that every interaction in life helps us gain a clear understanding of what we like, what we don't, what we will put up with, and most importantly, what we won't.
- Taking time out to be by ourselves is how we gain more clarity about ourselves.
- Remember that it takes a split second for words to leave our mouths but that they can live in a person's heart for a lifetime. Before speaking, ask yourself, "Is your need to say it greater than the other person's need to hear it?"

TRUST

Trust attunes our hearts and minds so that we can strengthen self belief and develop spontaneity, creativity and adventure in our lives.

- Listen to your feelings and let them guide you.
- Remember that feelings are more important than looks.
- Believe in everything you are and trust that it will take you to some greater good.
- Never ask of others what you would not joyfully do yourself.
- Open your heart first to yourself before you open it to someone else.
- Remain faithful to your gut feelings, even in the face of other people's logic.
- Accepting life with an attitude of calm strengthens trust.
- We can never trust ourselves too much, but we will live in fear if we don't.
- Put your heart into everything you do and remain true to yourself.

YOU

Your face is a faithful companion that is with you for life and needs to be honoured.

You sleep with it… so show it respect

You wear your troubles on it… so give it rest

You express yourself with it… so show it appreciation

You cry on it… so nurture it

You criticise it… so give it acceptance

You live and laugh with it… so love it!

Life is your party, celebrate it.
Live by your truth and leave the past behind.
Forgive with your heart not your head.
Laugh deliciously and feel what you feel
so you can heal.

But above all, remember there are no mistakes in life, only lessons that help us get clear about who we are, what we want and more importantly what we don't.

So never regret anything that made
you laugh or cry.

After all tears are drops of love that soften the heart and make love welcome, helping us to remember…

'That a face full of beauty is a
heart full of love'

FACE VALUE

SOME OF THE MOST POWERFUL ANTI-AGING PRODUCTS IN EXPENSIVE BEAUTY CREAMS CAN BE FOUND IN YOUR OWN KITCHEN!

FACE VALUE is jam packed with simple DIY secrets to beauty and great skin that achieve powerful results in a very short time.

Find out how the simple grape can eliminate fine lines or vinegar can restore the natural pH balance of your skin with the recipes in this powerful book.

Utilising natural ingredients full of skin regenerating Alpha Hydroxy Acid and Retin A, Collagen producing Vitamin C, skin healing Vitamin E and potent skin protecting antioxidants, **FACE VALUE** provides real solutions that target our greatest skin concerns.

Find recipes to…

- Reduce fine lines and wrinkles
- Stimulate collagen production
- Improve skin firmness and elasticity
- Protect skin from damaging free radicals
- Rehydrate, tighten and tone the face
- Restore the skin's radiance and natural pH levels
- Reduce age spots, pigmentation and blemishes

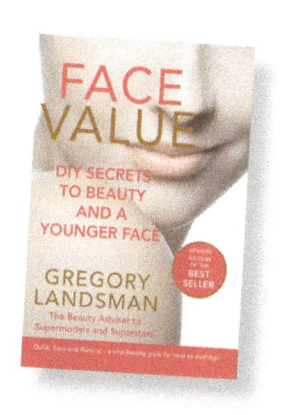

With **FACE VALUE**, you can achieve younger looking skin without having to leave your own kitchen!

Looking after your skin has never been simpler or more cost effective!

FACE LIFTING FOOD APPS

STOP FOOD AGING YOUR SKIN & EAT YOUR WAY TO YOUNGER, HEALTHIER LOOKING SKIN!

THE MOST POWERFUL ANTI-AGING INGREDIENTS CAN BE FOUND IN THE FOODS WE EAT. FACE LIFTING FOOD IS FULL OF EASY TO MAKE RECIPES WITH FOOD SECRETS THAT SUPPORT TIGHTER, BRIGHTER, YOUNGER LOOKING SKIN.

FACE LIFTING FOOD APPS feature easy to make recipes, revealing the most important natural foods full of powerful age defying vitamins and minerals that are essential to nurturing and protecting your skin's collagen which keeps the skin firm and elastic.

Optimise the health of your skin with recipes to:

- Counteract the aging process
- Stimulate and protect collagen
- Tighten skin and improve elasticity
- Reduce fine lines and wrinkles
- Protect skin with natural antioxidants
- Increase the thickness, and suppleness of skin
- Restore skin radiance

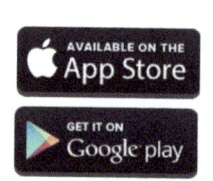

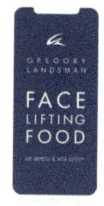

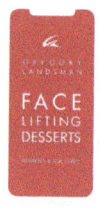

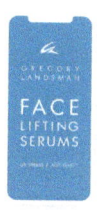

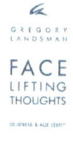

Attaining youthful looking skin has never been more simple or effective.

FACE FITNESS

FACE SECRETS

FACE SECRETS shows us how stress and daily living impacts our skin and provides 100% natural solutions to help keep skin strong and healthy.

In the book you will find formulas to help:

- Reduce fine lines
- Stimulate collagen and restore skin radiance
- Counteract the impact of stress and toxins that age the skin
- Activate youth enhancing hormones
- Plump out forehead worry lines
- Discover anti-aging foods

FACE LIFTING FOOD SKIN TREATMENTS

Gregory Landsman DIY Skin Treatment Prescriptives - real solutions to real skin challenges - dry skin; lip lines; dull skin; or problem skin. Transform your skin and take years off your face naturally!

gregorylandsmantreatments.com

STRESS FREE LIVING PODCAST

Listen to the STRESS FREE LIVING podcast with Gregory Landsman as he shares powerful stories about living your best life.

gregorylandsmanpodcast.com

FAITH LIFTING PRAYERS

Faith Lifting Prayers is a joyous celebration of our humanity and the beauty our individual differences bring to the world.

More than 20 years after writing the internationally acclaimed book, The Balance Of Beauty Explodes The Body Myth, Gregory brings us the follow up book, Faith Lifting Prayers, a compilation of the author's own stories and prayers written along his journey to find peace, fulfillment and a happy life.

Having grown up in South Africa under the Apartheid system, Gregory's early years were marked by daily beatings, bullying and rejection.

Sharing anecdotes that take us across the globe from South Africa to India, and from Switzerland to Australia, Gregory recounts incidents of humour and sadness that deliver a heartfelt reminder about the power of faith and the endurance of the human spirit.

Faith Lifting Prayers is a thought provoking and uplifting read to nourish the heart, lighten the spirit and inspire us to live our best lives.

"These prayers reflect back to us the beauty that shines within all of us, as we are all made in God's image."

Judith Durham AO, OAM, Singer

"I have treasured these prayers. The contemplation of just one prayer a day can bring peace and joy to your life as it did mine."

Yvette Grady, Four-time Emmy Award winning producer FOX, USA.

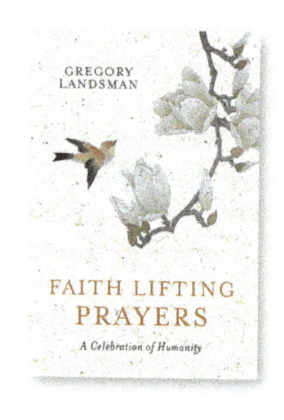

A LIFETIME OF BEAUTY

A Lifetime of Beauty is a story for parents to share with their children about what it takes to live a beautiful life.

Focussing on the power of individuality, A Lifetime of Beauty shines a light on the beauty in diversity and the richness each person's differences bring.

A Lifetime of Beauty is a wonderful reminder that for a child to build a strong foundation of self belief, self confidence and self worth, they must first believe in themselves and the spirit of their uniqueness.

A Lifetime of Beauty is a story that will warm your heart and can be shared with the whole family.

"We are all looking for true acceptance of ourselves physically, mentally and spiritually. The challenge for many is that since childhood, we are constantly being told or asked to change to fit in. We lose ourselves in the process and it often takes years to find ourselves again. The search is well worth it and essential to finding inner peace and true acceptance of ourselves and others. Gregory Landsman's transformational philosophy that underpins this book, helps guide us in this quest."

Dr Candy Aubry, child psychiatrist, psychoanalyst and ADHD specialist, Geneva, Switzerland

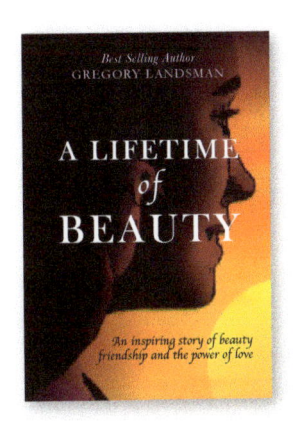

alifetimeofbeauty.com

Lightning Source UK Ltd.
Milton Keynes UK
UKHW020459270721
387798UK00007B/699